Medical Guide to Managing Chronic Fatigue and Fibromyalgia:

A Roadmap to Relief

"Prevention is better than cure."

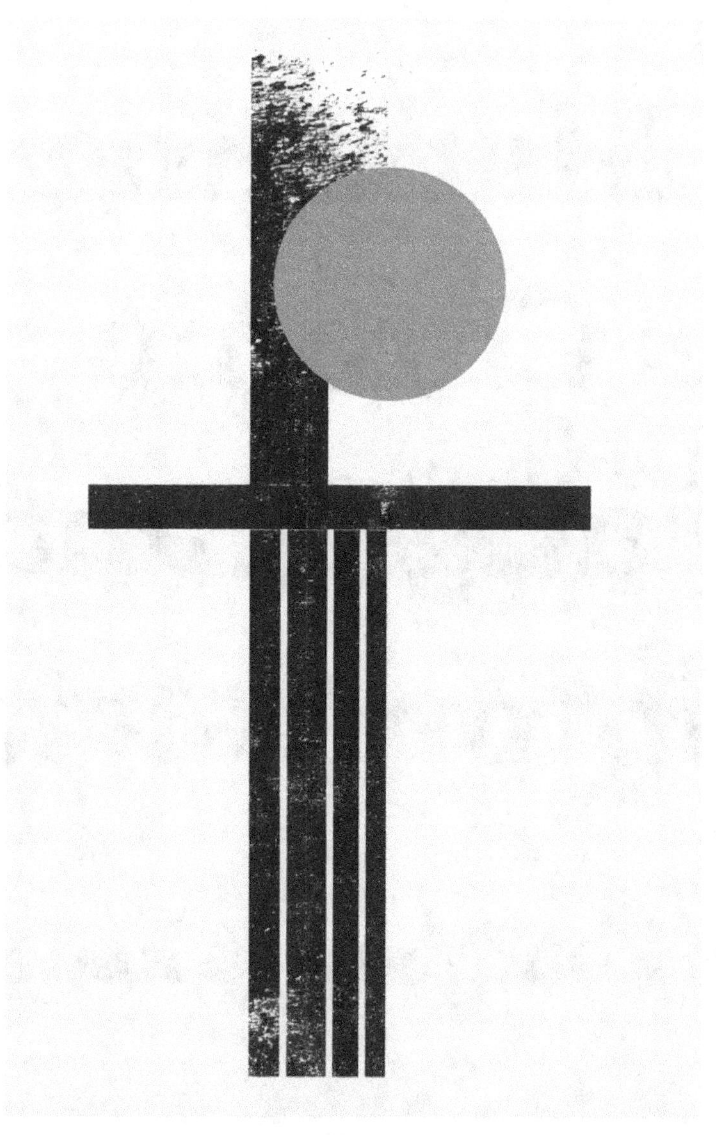

Introduction

Chronic fatigue and fibromyalgia can be overwhelming, but you don't have to navigate this journey alone. Medical Guide to Managing Chronic Fatigue and Fibromyalgia: A Roadmap to Relief offers a beacon of hope and a practical guide to reclaiming your life.

Discover evidence-based strategies, personalized treatment plans, and invaluable support as you embark on a path to renewed vitality. This book empowers you with the knowledge and tools to manage your symptoms, boost your energy levels, and experience a higher quality of life.

Let this book be your trusted companion as you rediscover your strength and embrace a brighter future.

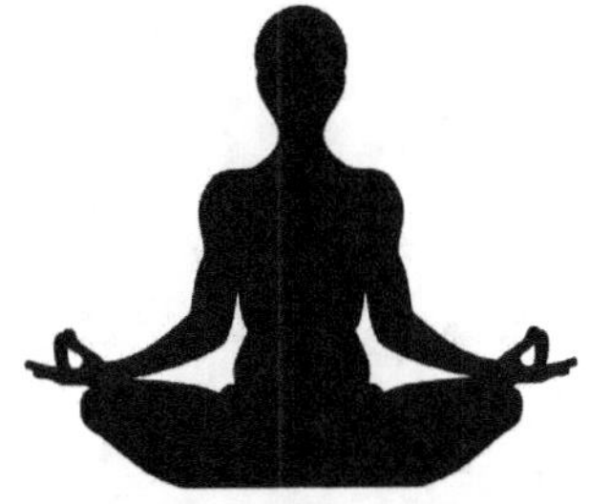

Contents

Contents

Contents

Contents

Part I: Understanding Chronic Fatigue and Fibromyalgia

Part I: Understanding Chronic Fatigue and Fibromyalgia
Chapter 1: Understanding Chronic Fatigue Syndrome (CFS)
1.1- Definition and Symptoms

Chronic Fatigue Syndrome (CFS), also known as Myalgic Encephalomyelitis (ME), is a complex disorder characterized by overwhelming fatigue that persists for at least six months and cannot be explained by an underlying medical condition. This fatigue significantly interferes with daily activities and doesn't improve with rest.

Symptoms

While fatigue is the hallmark symptom, CFS often involves a range of other debilitating symptoms. These can include:

- **Post-exertional malaise (PEM):** Worsening of symptoms after physical or mental exertion.
- **Unrefreshing sleep:** Difficulty sleeping, waking up feeling unrested, or excessive sleep without feeling refreshed.
- **Cognitive difficulties:** Problems with memory, concentration, and thinking, often referred to as "brain fog."
- **Muscle or joint pain:** Aching muscles and tender points.
- **Headaches:** Frequent or severe headaches.
- **Dizziness:** Feeling lightheaded or unsteady.
- **Sore throat:** Persistent or recurrent sore throat.
- **Enlarged lymph nodes:** Swollen lymph nodes in the neck or armpits.

It's important to note that the severity of symptoms can vary widely among individuals.

Part I: Understanding Chronic Fatigue and Fibromyalgia
Chapter 1: Understanding Chronic Fatigue Syndrome (CFS)
1.2- Prevalence and Impact

Prevalence

Determining the exact prevalence of Chronic Fatigue Syndrome (CFS) is challenging due to several factors, including:

- **Underdiagnosis:** Many cases of CFS go undiagnosed or misdiagnosed.

- **Varying diagnostic criteria:** Different criteria for diagnosing CFS can lead to inconsistent prevalence rates.

- **Lack of standardized assessment tools:** There is no universally accepted test for CFS, making it difficult to accurately identify cases.

Despite these challenges, studies suggest that CFS affects a significant number of people worldwide. While estimates vary, it's generally believed that CFS is more common in women than men.

Part I: Understanding Chronic Fatigue and Fibromyalgia
Chapter 1: Understanding Chronic Fatigue Syndrome (CFS)
1.2- Prevalence and Impact

Impact

The impact of CFS on individuals and society is substantial. People with CFS often experience significant limitations in their daily lives, including:

- Reduced quality of life: The constant fatigue and other symptoms can significantly impair a person's ability to participate in social, occupational, and recreational activities.

- Economic burden: CFS can lead to job loss, decreased productivity, and increased healthcare costs.

- Psychological distress: The chronic nature of CFS can contribute to depression, anxiety, and other mental health issues.

- Social isolation: As symptoms worsen, individuals with CFS may withdraw from social interactions, leading to feelings of loneliness and isolation.

It's essential to recognize the significant burden that CFS places on individuals and their families, as well as the broader economic and social implications of this condition.

Part I: Understanding Chronic Fatigue and Fibromyalgia
Chapter 1: Understanding Chronic Fatigue Syndrome (CFS)
1.3- The Difference Between CFS and Chronic Fatigue

Chronic fatigue is a general term used to describe persistent tiredness. It's a common symptom that can be caused by various factors such as stress, lack of sleep, poor diet, or underlying medical conditions.

Chronic Fatigue Syndrome (CFS), on the other hand, is a specific medical condition characterized by severe, debilitating fatigue that lasts for six months or more and cannot be explained by any underlying medical condition. CFS is accompanied by a range of other symptoms, such as post-exertional malaise (PEM), unrefreshing sleep, cognitive difficulties, and muscle or joint pain.

Key differences:

- Severity: CFS involves a much more severe and persistent level of fatigue than general chronic fatigue.

- Impact on daily life: CFS significantly interferes with daily activities, while chronic fatigue may simply cause reduced energy levels.

- Accompanying symptoms: CFS is associated with a specific set of symptoms, whereas chronic fatigue is often a symptom of another underlying condition.

Part I: Understanding Chronic Fatigue and Fibromyalgia
Chapter 1: Understanding Chronic Fatigue Syndrome (CFS)
1.3- The Difference Between CFS and Chronic Fatigue

It's important to note that while chronic fatigue can be a symptom of CFS, not all cases of chronic fatigue are CFS. If you're experiencing persistent and debilitating fatigue, it's essential to consult with a healthcare professional to determine the underlying cause.

Part I: Understanding Chronic Fatigue and Fibromyalgia
Chapter 2: Understanding Fibromyalgia
2.1- Definition and Symptoms

Definition

Fibromyalgia is a chronic condition characterized by widespread musculoskeletal pain accompanied by fatigue, sleep disturbances, memory and mood issues. It's believed to amplify pain signals, affecting how the brain processes pain.

Symptoms

- **Widespread pain**: A constant dull ache often described as feeling like a body-wide sunburn.
- **Fatigue:** Persistent tiredness, even after adequate sleep.
- **Sleep disturbances**: Difficulty falling asleep, staying asleep, or feeling unrefreshed upon waking.
- **Cognitive difficulties**: Problems with memory, concentration, and focus, often referred to as "fibro fog."
- **Mood disorders**: Anxiety, depression, and irritability are common.
- **Headaches:** Frequent or severe headaches.
- **Irritable bowel syndrome (IBS)**: Digestive issues such as bloating, constipation, or diarrhea.

It's important to note that symptoms can vary in intensity and frequency among individuals.

Part I: Understanding Chronic Fatigue and Fibromyalgia
Chapter 2: Understanding Fibromyalgia
2.2- Prevalence and Impact

Prevalence

Fibromyalgia is a relatively common condition, affecting an estimated 2-4% of the general population. It is significantly more prevalent in women than in men. The exact prevalence can vary depending on factors such as age, geographic location, and diagnostic criteria.

Impact

Fibromyalgia can have a profound impact on a person's quality of life. The chronic pain, fatigue, and other symptoms associated with the condition can interfere with daily activities, work, and social interactions.

- Physical limitations: The widespread pain and fatigue can make it difficult to perform even simple tasks.

- Psychological impact: Fibromyalgia often co-occurs with conditions like depression, anxiety, and irritable bowel syndrome, further impacting mental health and well-being.

- Social isolation: Due to the challenges posed by the condition, individuals with fibromyalgia may withdraw from social activities, leading to feelings of loneliness and isolation.

- Economic burden: The condition can result in job loss, decreased productivity, and increased healthcare costs.

Part I: Understanding Chronic Fatigue and Fibromyalgia
Chapter 2: Understanding Fibromyalgia
2.2- Prevalence and Impact

It's important to recognize the significant challenges faced by individuals with fibromyalgia and the need for comprehensive support and treatment.

Part I: Understanding Chronic Fatigue and Fibromyalgia
Chapter 2: Understanding Fibromyalgia
2.3- The Relationship Between CFS and Fibromyalgia

The relationship between Chronic Fatigue Syndrome (CFS) and Fibromyalgia is complex and often debated among medical professionals.

Overlapping Symptoms

One of the most striking aspects of these two conditions is the significant overlap in their symptoms. Both involve:

- Chronic fatigue: A persistent and debilitating tiredness.

- Pain: While fibromyalgia is primarily characterized by widespread musculoskeletal pain, many individuals with CFS also experience pain.

- Sleep disturbances: Difficulty falling asleep, staying asleep, or feeling unrefreshed upon waking.

- Cognitive difficulties: Problems with memory, concentration, and focus.

Due to these shared symptoms, it's not uncommon for individuals to be diagnosed with both CFS and fibromyalgia.
Distinct Conditions

Part I: Understanding Chronic Fatigue and Fibromyalgia
Chapter 2: Understanding Fibromyalgia
2.3- The Relationship Between CFS and Fibromyalgia

Despite the overlapping symptoms, CFS and fibromyalgia are considered distinct conditions. Some key differences include:

- Primary symptom: Fatigue is the primary symptom of CFS, while pain is the primary symptom of fibromyalgia.

- Post-exertional malaise (PEM): This is a hallmark symptom of CFS, but it's less common in fibromyalgia.

- Underlying mechanisms: While both conditions involve dysregulation of the nervous system, the specific mechanisms are believed to differ.

The Debate Continues

The exact relationship between CFS and fibromyalgia is still under investigation. Some experts believe they are separate conditions with overlapping symptoms, while others suggest they may be different manifestations of the same underlying disorder.

It's important to note that having one condition does not automatically mean you will develop the other. However, the high rate of comorbidity (both conditions occurring together) highlights the need for further research to better understand the connection between these two complex conditions.

Part I: Understanding Chronic Fatigue and Fibromyalgia
Chapter 3: The Roots of Chronic Fatigue and Fibromyalgia
3.1- Potential Causes and Triggers

Disclaimer: While research has made progress, the exact causes of Chronic Fatigue Syndrome (CFS) and Fibromyalgia remain elusive. The following information outlines potential factors and triggers based on current understanding.

Potential Causes and Triggers

While the precise causes of CFS and fibromyalgia are unknown, several factors are believed to contribute to their development:

Genetic Predisposition

- Inherited traits: Some individuals may have a genetic susceptibility to developing these conditions.

- Family history: A family history of CFS, fibromyalgia, or related conditions can increase the risk.

Immune System Dysfunction

- Viral infections: Some research suggests that viral infections may trigger or contribute to the development of CFS.

- Autoimmune disorders: There is evidence linking CFS and fibromyalgia to autoimmune conditions.

Part I: Understanding Chronic Fatigue and Fibromyalgia
Chapter 3: The Roots of Chronic Fatigue and Fibromyalgia
3.1- Potential Causes and Triggers

Neurological Factors

- Central nervous system abnormalities: Dysregulation of the nervous system may play a role in both conditions.

- Pain processing: Fibromyalgia is associated with amplified pain signals, suggesting abnormal pain processing in the brain.

Environmental Factors

- Stress: Psychological and physical stress can exacerbate symptoms and potentially contribute to the development of CFS and fibromyalgia.

- Toxins: Exposure to certain chemicals or environmental toxins may be linked to these conditions.

- Sleep disturbances: Sleep problems can worsen symptoms and may be a contributing factor.

Hormonal Factors

- Hormonal imbalances: Fluctuations in hormones, particularly in women, may influence the development or severity of symptoms.

Part I: Understanding Chronic Fatigue and Fibromyalgia
Chapter 3: The Roots of Chronic Fatigue and Fibromyalgia
3.1- Potential Causes and Triggers

It's important to emphasize that these are potential factors and the exact cause of CFS and fibromyalgia often remains unclear. Many individuals may experience a combination of these factors.

The Role of the Immune System in Chronic Fatigue Syndrome (CFS) and Fibromyalgia

The immune system plays a significant role in both Chronic Fatigue Syndrome (CFS) and Fibromyalgia. While the exact mechanisms are still being studied, there's growing evidence suggesting abnormalities in immune function contribute to these conditions.

Immune System Dysfunction in CFS

- Chronic activation: The immune system may be in a state of chronic activation, leading to persistent inflammation.

- Viral persistence: Some research suggests that certain viruses may trigger or contribute to CFS by persisting in the body and causing ongoing immune activation.

- Autoimmune-like features: In some cases, CFS may share characteristics with autoimmune diseases, suggesting potential immune system dysregulation.

Immune System Dysfunction in Fibromyalgia

- Increased inflammation: Studies have shown elevated levels of inflammatory markers in people with fibromyalgia.

Part I: Understanding Chronic Fatigue and Fibromyalgia
Chapter 3: The Roots of Chronic Fatigue and Fibromyalgia
3.2- The Role of the Immune System

- Abnormal immune response: The immune system may be overreacting to stimuli, contributing to pain and fatigue.

- Autoimmune connection: There's evidence suggesting a potential link between fibromyalgia and autoimmune diseases, indicating possible immune system involvement.

Key points:

- Both CFS and fibromyalgia involve immune system abnormalities, although the specific mechanisms differ.

- Chronic inflammation is a common feature in both conditions.

- Research is ongoing to better understand the complex interplay between the immune system and these conditions.

Part I: Understanding Chronic Fatigue and Fibromyalgia
Chapter 3: The Roots of Chronic Fatigue and Fibromyalgia
3.3- Genetic and Environmental Factors

While research is ongoing, there is increasing evidence suggesting a genetic component to both Chronic Fatigue Syndrome (CFS) and Fibromyalgia.

- Family history: A family history of these conditions or related disorders can increase the risk.

- Genetic markers: Researchers are studying specific genes that may be linked to these conditions.

- Twin studies: Studies of identical twins have shown higher rates of concordance for CFS and fibromyalgia, suggesting a genetic influence.

It's important to note that having a genetic predisposition does not guarantee developing the condition. Other factors, such as environmental triggers, also play a role.

Environmental Factors

Environmental factors can interact with genetic susceptibility to influence the development of CFS and fibromyalgia. Some potential environmental triggers include:

- Infections: Viral infections, such as Epstein-Barr virus (EBV), have been associated with CFS.

- Toxins: Exposure to certain chemicals or environmental pollutants may contribute to symptom development.

3.3- Genetic and Environmental Factors

- Stress: Psychological and physical stress can exacerbate symptoms and potentially trigger the onset of these conditions.

- Trauma: Physical or emotional trauma may be associated with an increased risk.

- Sleep disturbances: Chronic sleep deprivation can worsen symptoms and may be a contributing factor.

It's essential to consider the complex interplay between genetic and environmental factors in understanding the development of CFS and fibromyalgia.

Part II: Conventional and Complementary Treatments

4.1- Current Treatment Options

there are no specific cures for Chronic Fatigue Syndrome (CFS) or Fibromyalgia. However, a combination of medical treatments, lifestyle modifications, and complementary therapies can help manage symptoms and improve quality of life.

Current Treatment Options

Note: Treatment approaches are often tailored to individual needs and symptom severity.

Medications

- Pain relievers: Over-the-counter or prescription medications can help manage pain.

- Antidepressants: Some antidepressants, such as duloxetine and milnacipran, are approved for fibromyalgia and may also help with fatigue.

- Anti-seizure medications: Drugs like gabapentin and pregabalin can be effective in managing pain and sleep disturbances.

- Sleep aids: Prescription sleep medications may be used to address severe sleep problems.

4.1- Current Treatment Options

Lifestyle Modifications

- Graded exercise therapy: Gradually increasing physical activity can improve energy levels and reduce pain.

- Cognitive-behavioral therapy (CBT): This therapy helps manage pain, fatigue, and other symptoms by addressing thoughts and behaviors.

- Sleep hygiene: Establishing good sleep habits can improve sleep quality.

- Stress management: Techniques like meditation, yoga, or deep breathing can help reduce stress.

- Pacing activities: Balancing rest and activity is essential for managing energy levels.

Complementary Therapies

- Acupuncture: May help with pain and fatigue.
- Massage therapy: Can relax muscles and reduce pain.
- Chiropractic care: May improve spinal alignment and reduce pain.

4.1- Current Treatment Options

Challenges in Treatment

- Lack of specific treatments: There is no one-size-fits-all approach for CFS or fibromyalgia.

- Symptom variability: Symptoms can fluctuate, making treatment challenging.

- Patient variability: Individuals respond differently to treatments.

It's essential to work closely with healthcare providers to develop a personalized treatment plan. While there's no cure, many people with CFS and fibromyalgia can experience significant improvements in their quality of life with appropriate management.

4.2- Medication and Their Uses

While there's no specific cure for CFS or Fibromyalgia, medications can help manage symptoms. It's essential to consult with a healthcare provider for personalized treatment plans.

Pain Relievers

- Over-the-counter (OTC) pain relievers: Medications like ibuprofen, naproxen, or acetaminophen can help manage mild to moderate pain.

- Prescription pain relievers: For more severe pain, doctors may prescribe stronger pain relievers.

Antidepressants

- Duloxetine and milnacipran: These medications are approved for fibromyalgia and can help with pain, fatigue, and sleep disturbances.

- Other antidepressants: In some cases, other antidepressants might be used to address mood symptoms associated with CFS and fibromyalgia.

Anti-seizure Medications

- Gabapentin and pregabalin: These drugs can help manage nerve pain and improve sleep quality.

Sleep Aids

- Prescription sleep medications: For severe sleep disturbances, doctors may prescribe sleep aids.

Important Considerations

- Side effects: All medications have potential side effects. It's crucial to weigh the benefits against the risks.

- Combination therapy: Often, a combination of medications and non-pharmacological treatments works best.

- Regular monitoring: Regular check-ups with your doctor are essential to monitor medication effectiveness and adjust treatment as needed.

Please note: This information is for general knowledge and doesn't replace professional medical advice. Always consult with a healthcare provider for diagnosis and treatment.

4.3- Role of Healthcare Providers

Healthcare providers play a crucial role in diagnosing, managing, and supporting individuals with Chronic Fatigue Syndrome (CFS) and Fibromyalgia.

Diagnostic Role

- Comprehensive evaluation: Healthcare providers conduct thorough medical histories, physical examinations, and often order tests to rule out other potential causes of symptoms.

- Symptom assessment: Careful evaluation of symptoms is essential to differentiate between CFS, fibromyalgia, and other conditions.

Treatment Planning

- Personalized approach: Healthcare providers develop individualized treatment plans based on a patient's specific symptoms and needs.

- Medication management: Prescribing appropriate medications to manage pain, fatigue, and other symptoms.

- Lifestyle recommendations: Providing guidance on pacing activities, sleep hygiene, stress management, and diet.

4.3- Role of Healthcare Providers

- Referrals: Referring patients to specialists, such as pain management specialists, mental health professionals, or physical therapists, when necessary.

Patient Education and Support

- Understanding the conditions: Providing information about CFS and fibromyalgia, including causes, symptoms, and treatment options.

- Coping strategies: Offering guidance on coping with the challenges of living with chronic illness.

- Emotional support: Providing emotional support and encouragement.

Ongoing Monitoring

- Regular check-ups: Monitoring patients' progress and adjusting treatment plans as needed.

- Symptom management: Helping patients manage symptom flares and develop coping mechanisms.

It's important to find a healthcare provider who understands CFS and fibromyalgia and is committed to providing comprehensive care. Building a strong patient-provider relationship is essential for effective management of these conditions.

Pacing is a cornerstone of managing Chronic Fatigue Syndrome (CFS) and Fibromyalgia. It involves carefully balancing activity and rest to prevent symptom exacerbation.

Understanding Your Energy Levels

- Identify your baseline: Determine your current energy level and recognize your limitations.

- Track your activities: Keep a journal to monitor how different activities impact your energy.

- Listen to your body: Pay attention to your body's signals and avoid pushing yourself beyond your limits.

Energy Conservation Techniques

- Prioritize tasks: Focus on essential activities and delegate or eliminate less important ones.

- Break down tasks: Divide larger tasks into smaller, manageable steps.

- Rest frequently: Incorporate short rest periods throughout the day.

- Build-in flexibility: Allow for adjustments in your schedule based on how you feel.

- Set realistic goals: Avoid overcommitting and setting unrealistic expectations.

Avoiding Overexertion

- Pace yourself: Gradually increase activity levels, avoiding sudden bursts of energy expenditure.

- Recognize your limits: Learn to say no to additional responsibilities when necessary.

- Plan ahead: Anticipate energy demands and plan accordingly.

Energy Envelope

The concept of an "energy envelope" can be helpful. Imagine your energy level as a container with a limited capacity. Activities fill this container. If you overfill it, you'll experience a crash. The goal is to find a balance that allows you to function without depleting your energy reserves.
By implementing these strategies, individuals with CFS and fibromyalgia can improve their ability to manage daily activities and reduce symptom severity.

Healthy Sleep Habits for CFS and Fibromyalgia
Sleep is crucial for recovery and energy restoration in individuals with Chronic Fatigue Syndrome (CFS) and Fibromyalgia. Establishing healthy sleep habits can significantly improve your overall well-being.

Creating a Sleep-Conducive Environment

- Dark, quiet, and cool: Ensure your bedroom is a peaceful sanctuary.

- Comfortable bedding: Invest in a comfortable mattress, pillows, and bedding.

- Limit screen time: Avoid electronic devices at least an hour before bed.

- Create a relaxing bedtime routine: Engage in calming activities like reading or taking a warm bath.

Sleep Hygiene Practices

- Consistent sleep schedule: Go to bed and wake up at the same time every day, even on weekends.

- Limit daytime naps: While short naps can be beneficial, excessive napping can disrupt nighttime sleep.

- Regular exercise: Engage in physical activity, but avoid intense workouts close to bedtime.

- Manage stress: Practice relaxation techniques like meditation or deep breathing.

- Limit caffeine and alcohol: Reduce consumption of caffeine and alcohol, especially close to bedtime.

- Watch your diet: Avoid heavy meals close to bedtime.

Addressing Sleep Disruptions

- Sleep aids: If sleep problems persist, consult your doctor about potential sleep aids.

- Sleep studies: In some cases, a sleep study may be necessary to identify underlying sleep disorders.

By prioritizing sleep and implementing these strategies, you can significantly improve your sleep quality and overall well-being.

Stress can significantly exacerbate symptoms of Chronic Fatigue Syndrome (CFS) and Fibromyalgia. Incorporating stress reduction techniques into your daily routine can help improve your overall well-being.

Relaxation Techniques

- Deep breathing: Focus on slow, deep breaths to calm the mind and body.

- Progressive muscle relaxation: Tense and relax different muscle groups to release physical tension.

- Meditation and mindfulness: Cultivate present-moment awareness and reduce stress.

- Yoga and tai chi: Gentle forms of exercise that combine physical movement with mental focus.

Lifestyle Modifications

- Time management: Prioritize tasks and avoid overcommitting.

- Setting boundaries: Learn to say no to additional responsibilities when needed.

- Spending time in nature: Connect with the outdoors to reduce stress and improve mood.

- Hobbies and interests: Engage in activities you enjoy to promote relaxation and enjoyment.

Support Systems

- Social connections: Maintain strong relationships with friends and family.

- Support groups: Connect with others who understand your condition.

- Professional help: Consider therapy or counseling to address emotional challenges.

Remember, it's essential to find stress reduction techniques that work best for you. Start with small steps and gradually incorporate more techniques into your routine.

General Dietary Principles

- Focus on whole foods: Prioritize fruits, vegetables, whole grains, lean proteins, and healthy fats.

- Hydration: Drink plenty of water throughout the day.

- Portion control: Be mindful of portion sizes to avoid feeling overwhelmed.

- Regular meals: Aim for regular meal times to stabilize blood sugar levels.

- Limit processed foods: Reduce intake of processed foods, sugary drinks, and excessive caffeine.

Nutrients to Consider

- Antioxidants: Found in fruits, vegetables, and nuts, antioxidants help combat oxidative stress.

- Omega-3 fatty acids: Found in fatty fish, flaxseed, and chia seeds, they may help reduce inflammation.

- Magnesium: Essential for muscle and nerve function, found in leafy green vegetables, nuts, and seeds.

Potential Dietary Triggers

- Food sensitivities: Some individuals with CFS or Fibromyalgia report improvements after eliminating certain foods, such as gluten, dairy, or caffeine.

- Blood sugar fluctuations: Unstable blood sugar levels can contribute to fatigue.

Important Considerations

- Individual variations: Nutritional needs vary from person to person.

- Consulting a healthcare professional: Consider consulting a registered dietitian for personalized guidance.

- Food journaling: Tracking your food intake can help identify potential triggers or nutritional deficiencies.

By adopting a healthy and balanced diet, you can provide your body with the necessary nutrients to support overall well-being and potentially improve symptoms of CFS andFibromyalgia.

Consuming nutrient-rich foods can help boost energy levels and support overall well-being. Here are some excellent options:

Complex Carbohydrates

These provide sustained energy and help stabilize blood sugar levels.

- Whole grains: Brown rice, quinoa, oats, whole-wheat bread
- Legumes: Lentils, chickpeas, beans
- Sweet potatoes and other starchy vegetables

Lean Proteins

Essential for building and repairing tissues, proteins also contribute to satiety.

- Poultry: Chicken, turkey
- Fish: Salmon, tuna, mackerel
- Eggs
- Legumes: Lentils, chickpeas, beans
- Tofu and tempeh

Healthy Fats

These provide energy and support nutrient absorption.

- Avocados
- Nuts and seeds: Almonds, walnuts, chia seeds, flaxseeds
- Olive oil

Fruits and Vegetables

Packed with vitamins, minerals, and antioxidants.

- Berries: Blueberries, raspberries, strawberries
- Leafy greens: Spinach, kale, collard greens
- Citrus fruits: Oranges, grapefruits
- Bell peppers

Additional Tips

- Hydration: Drink plenty of water throughout the day.
- Portion control: Avoid overeating to prevent energy crashes.
- Regular meals: Consuming balanced meals every few hours helps maintain stable energy levels.
- Limit processed foods: These often contain added sugars and unhealthy fats.

Remember: Individual needs vary. It's essential to listen to your body and find what works best for you. If you have specific dietary concerns or conditions, consult with a healthcare professional or registered dietitian.

Supplements and Their Benefits

Disclaimer: While supplements can be beneficial, it's crucial to consult with a healthcare provider before starting any new supplement regimen. They can provide personalized guidance and address potential interactions with medications.

Supplements can offer additional support for individuals with Chronic Fatigue Syndrome (CFS) and Fibromyalgia. Here are some commonly explored options:

Vitamins and Minerals

- Vitamin D: Essential for bone health, immune function, and mood regulation.

- Magnesium: Supports muscle relaxation, sleep, and energy production.

- B vitamins: Contribute to energy metabolism and nerve function.

- Iron: Essential for oxygen transport and energy production.

Other Supplements

- Coenzyme Q10 (CoQ10): Involved in energy production.
- Omega-3 fatty acids: May help reduce inflammation.
- SAMe (S-adenosyl-L-methionine): Shown to improve mood and reduce pain in some studies.
- Acetyl-L-carnitine: May help with energy production and cognitive function.

Potential Benefits

- Energy boost: Some supplements can help increase energy levels.

- Reduced inflammation: Certain supplements have anti-inflammatory properties.

- Improved sleep: Some supplements can promote better sleep quality.

- Pain management: Certain supplements may help alleviate pain.

Important Considerations

- Quality and dosage: Choose reputable brands and follow recommended dosages.

- Potential side effects: Be aware of potential side effects and interactions with medications.

- Individual variability: What works for one person may not work for another.

- Holistic approach: Supplements should be part of a comprehensive treatment plan, including diet, exercise, and stress management.

While it might seem counterintuitive, regular physical activity is crucial for managing Chronic Fatigue Syndrome (CFS) and Fibromyalgia.

Benefits of Exercise

- Increased energy: Regular exercise can paradoxically boost energy levels.

- Pain reduction: Physical activity can help alleviate chronic pain.

- Improved mood: Exercise is a natural mood enhancer, helping to combat depression and anxiety often associated with CFS and Fibromyalgia.

- Better sleep: Regular physical activity can improve sleep quality.

- Strengthened muscles and bones: Exercise helps build and maintain muscle and bone strength.

- Enhanced overall health: Regular physical activity supports overall health and well-being.

It's essential to approach exercise gradually and listen to your body. Overexertion can lead to symptom flare-ups.

The key to successful exercise for individuals with CFS and Fibromyalgia is to start slowly, listen to your body, and gradually increase activity levels.

Low-Impact Exercise Options:

- Walking: Begin with short walks and gradually increase distance and pace.

- Swimming: The buoyancy of water reduces joint stress.

- Cycling: Stationary or outdoor cycling can be a low-impact option.

- Yoga and Tai Chi: These gentle practices improve flexibility, balance, and relaxation.

- Water aerobics: Provides a low-impact workout with the added benefits of water resistance.

Strength Training:

- Light weights: Focus on building strength gradually with light weights or resistance bands.

- Bodyweight exercises: Exercises like squats, lunges, and push-ups can be modified to suit your fitness level.

Important Considerations:

- Gradual progression: Start with short exercise sessions and gradually increase duration and intensity.

- Listen to your body: Pay attention to your body's signals and rest when needed.

- Warm-up and cool-down: Incorporate stretching and gentle movements before and after exercise.

- Variety: Incorporate different types of exercise to prevent boredom and plateaus.

- Professional guidance: Consider working with a physical therapist or exercise specialist for personalized guidance.

Remember: It's essential to find an exercise routine that works for you. What works for one person may not work for another. Be patient and persistent, and celebrate small victories along the way.

Understanding the Importance of Gradual Progression
When starting an exercise program for Chronic Fatigue
Syndrome (CFS) or Fibromyalgia, it's crucial to increase
activity levels gradually. This prevents overexertion, which
can lead to symptom flare-ups and setbacks.

Key Principles:

- Start slow: Begin with very short exercise sessions, even if
  it's just a few minutes.

- Listen to your body: Pay close attention to your body's
  signals. If you experience excessive fatigue or pain, reduce
  the intensity or duration of your exercise.

- Consistency: Regular, low-intensity exercise is more
  beneficial than sporadic high-intensity workouts.

- Variety: Incorporate different types of exercise to prevent
  boredom and plateaus.

Example of a Gradual Increase Plan:

- Week 1: Start with 5 minutes of light walking or gentle
  stretching.
- Week 2: Increase to 7 minutes of walking or stretching.
- Week 3: Add 2-3 minutes of light strength training
  exercises.
- Week 4: Increase walking or stretching to 10 minutes.

Remember: This is just a general guideline. Everyone's progress will be different. Be patient with yourself and celebrate small victories.

Additional Tips:

- Track your progress: Keep a journal to monitor your energy levels and exercise tolerance.

- Cross-training: Incorporate different types of exercise to prevent plateaus and reduce the risk of overuse injuries.

- Rest days: Schedule rest days to allow your body to recover.

- Flexibility: Be prepared to adjust your exercise routine based on how you feel.

Cognitive Behavioral Therapy (CBT) is a psychological treatment that has shown effectiveness in managing chronic pain conditions like Chronic Fatigue Syndrome (CFS) and Fibromyalgia. It focuses on the relationship between thoughts, feelings, and behaviors.

How CBT Helps

- Challenge negative thoughts: CBT helps individuals identify and challenge negative thought patterns that contribute to pain, fatigue, and low mood.

- Develop coping strategies: It teaches practical skills for managing symptoms, such as time management, pacing activities, and problem-solving.

- Improve sleep: CBT can address sleep disturbances, a common symptom of CFS and fibromyalgia.

- Enhance mood: By improving coping mechanisms and reducing negative thinking, CBT can help elevate mood.

CBT Techniques

- Identifying and challenging negative thoughts: Recognizing and replacing unhelpful thought patterns with more realistic and positive ones.

- Pacing activities: Learning to balance rest and activity to prevent symptom flare-ups.

- Sleep hygiene: Developing healthy sleep habits to improve sleep quality.

- Relaxation techniques: Incorporating relaxation methods like deep breathing, meditation, or progressive muscle relaxation.

Benefits of CBT

- Improved pain management
- Increased energy levels
- Enhanced mood and reduced anxiety
- Better sleep quality
- Improved overall quality of life

Managing pain is a significant challenge for individuals with Chronic Fatigue Syndrome (CFS) and Fibromyalgia. Here are some strategies that can help:

Physical Therapies

- Heat and cold therapy: Applying heat or cold packs to painful areas can provide temporary relief.

- Massage: Can help relax muscles and reduce pain.

- Physical therapy: A physical therapist can teach specific exercises and stretches to improve flexibility and strength.

Lifestyle Modifications

- Pacing activities: Avoiding overexertion can help prevent pain flare-ups.

- Ergonomics: Ensuring your workspace is ergonomically correct can reduce physical strain.

- Sleep hygiene: Prioritizing quality sleep can help manage pain.

Complementary Therapies

- Acupuncture: May help reduce pain and improve overall well-being.

- Yoga and Tai Chi: Gentle movements can help with pain management and relaxation.

- Mindfulness and meditation: These practices can help reduce stress and pain perception.

Medications

- Over-the-counter pain relievers: While not a long-term solution, they can provide temporary relief.

- Prescription medications: In some cases, doctors may prescribe medications specifically for pain management.

Remember: It's essential to work with your healthcare provider to find the most effective pain management strategies for you.

Living with Chronic Fatigue Syndrome (CFS) or Fibromyalgia can be emotionally challenging. Feelings of frustration, anger, sadness, and isolation are common. Here are some strategies to help manage these emotions:

Understanding Your Emotions

- Acknowledge your feelings: It's important to recognize and validate your emotions.

- Identify triggers: Understanding what situations or factors contribute to emotional distress can help you develop coping strategies.

- Practice self-compassion: Be kind to yourself and avoid self-blame.

Building Resilience

- Develop a support system: Connect with friends, family, or support groups who understand your condition.

- Set realistic goals: Focus on achievable goals to build a sense of accomplishment.

- Practice gratitude: Focusing on the positive aspects of your life can improve your mood.

- Time management: Effective time management can reduce stress and frustration.

Seeking Professional Help

- Therapy: A therapist can provide tools and strategies for managing emotional challenges.

- Counseling: Talking to a counselor can help you process your feelings and develop coping mechanisms.

Self-Care

- Mindfulness and meditation: These practices can help reduce stress and anxiety.

- Physical activity: Even gentle exercise can improve mood.

- Healthy lifestyle: Prioritize sleep, nutrition, and relaxation.

Remember, it's okay to seek help. You don't have to go through this alone.

Ayurveda, an ancient Indian system of medicine, offers a holistic approach to managing chronic fatigue. It focuses on balancing the body, mind, and spirit for optimal health.

Understanding the Three Doshas

Ayurveda recognizes three fundamental energies or doshas: Vata, Pitta, and Kapha. An imbalance in these doshas can lead to various health issues, including chronic fatigue.

- Vata: Governs movement, creativity, and energy. An imbalance can manifest as fatigue, anxiety, and digestive issues.

- Pitta: Related to metabolism, digestion, and transformation. Imbalance can lead to inflammation and irritability.

- Kapha: Associated with structure, stability, and immunity. An imbalance can result in sluggishness and weight gain.

Ayurvedic Principles for Managing Chronic Fatigue

- Individualized approach: Ayurveda emphasizes a personalized approach to healthcare, considering each individual's unique constitution.

- Balance: The goal is to restore balance to the doshas through diet, lifestyle, and herbal remedies.

- Holistic healing: Ayurveda addresses the whole person, considering physical, mental, and emotional well-being.

- Prevention: Ayurveda focuses on preventing disease through healthy lifestyle practices.

Ayurvedic Practices for Chronic Fatigue

- Diet: Consuming warm, nourishing foods that are easy to digest is crucial.

- Lifestyle: Regular routines, adequate sleep, and stress management are essential.

- Herbs: Ayurvedic herbs like Ashwagandha, Shatavari, and Amalaki can support energy levels.

- Panchakarma: This detoxification process can help restore balance to the body.

- Yoga and meditation: These practices promote relaxation and energy balance.

By understanding your unique dosha constitution and incorporating Ayurvedic principles into your daily life, you can effectively manage chronic fatigue and improve overall well-being.

Ayurveda emphasizes a personalized approach to healthcare, recognizing that each individual is unique. This principle is particularly important in managing chronic fatigue.

Assessing Individual Needs

Before creating a treatment plan, an Ayurvedic practitioner will conduct a comprehensive assessment, considering:

- Prakriti (constitution): Determining the dominant dosha (Vata, Pitta, or Kapha) to understand inherent strengths and weaknesses.

- Vikruti (imbalance): Assessing the current state of imbalance and its impact on the body.

- Digestive fire (Agni): Evaluating the strength of the digestive system, as it's crucial for energy production.

- Lifestyle factors: Considering factors like diet, sleep, stress, and occupation.

Tailored Treatment Plan

Based on the assessment, a customized treatment plan is developed, incorporating:

- Diet: Specific food recommendations based on the individual's dosha and digestive capacity.

- Lifestyle modifications: Tailored advice on sleep, exercise, and daily routines.

- Herbal remedies: Selecting herbs that address the root cause of fatigue and support overall well-being.

- Panchakarma (detoxification): Recommending specific Panchakarma therapies based on the individual's needs.

Example Treatment Plans

- Vata-dominant individual: Focus on grounding, warming foods, regular routines, and stress management.

- Pitta-dominant individual: Prioritize cooling, calming foods, and stress reduction techniques.

- Kapha-dominant individual: Emphasize stimulating foods, regular exercise, and lighter meals.

It's essential to consult with a qualified Ayurvedic practitioner to create a personalized treatment plan.

Ayurveda offers a range of herbs and supplements to address chronic fatigue. It's essential to consult with an Ayurvedic practitioner for personalized recommendations.

Adaptogenic Herbs

- Ashwagandha (Withania somnifera): Known as "Indian ginseng," Ashwagandha helps manage stress, improves sleep, and boosts energy levels.

- Ginseng (Panax ginseng): Enhances physical and mental performance, reduces fatigue, and supports the immune system.

- Rhodiola rosea: Adaptogenic herb that helps with fatigue, improves mood, and enhances cognitive function.

Digestive Support

- Triphala: A blend of three fruits, Triphala supports digestion, detoxification, and overall well-being.

- Amalaki (Indian gooseberry): Rich in vitamin C, Amalaki strengthens the immune system and improves digestion.

Other Ayurvedic Herbs

- Shatavari (Asparagus racemosus): Nourishes the reproductive system, supports hormonal balance, and helps with fatigue.

- Brahmi (Bacopa monnieri): Improves memory, focus, and reduces anxiety.

Important Considerations

- Quality and source: Choose high-quality herbs from reputable suppliers.

- Consultation: Consult with an Ayurvedic practitioner to determine the best herbs for your specific needs.

- Dosage: Follow recommended dosages and consult with a healthcare provider.

- Potential interactions: Inform your doctor about any herbs or supplements you're taking.

Remember: While herbs can be beneficial, they are not a substitute for medical treatment. It's essential to work with a healthcare provider to address underlying health issues.

Yoga offers a holistic approach to improving energy levels and overall well-being. It combines physical postures, breathing exercises, and meditation to balance the body and mind.

How Yoga Boosts Energy

- Increased circulation: Yoga poses stimulate blood flow, delivering oxygen and nutrients to the body's tissues.

- Improved flexibility: Regular practice enhances flexibility, reducing muscle tension and improving posture.

- Stress reduction: Yoga's calming effects help manage stress, a common energy drain.

- Enhanced focus: Meditation and breathing exercises improve concentration and mental clarity.

- Boosted immune system: Regular yoga practice can strengthen the immune system.

Yoga Poses for Energy

- Inversions: Poses like downward-facing dog and headstand increase blood flow to the brain, boosting energy.

- Standing poses: Warrior poses, triangle pose, and tree pose strengthen the legs and core, improving balance and stability.

- Backbends: Poses like cobra and camel pose open the chest and lungs, increasing oxygen intake.

Breathing Techniques (Pranayama)

- Nadi Shodhana (Alternate Nostril Breathing): Balances the energy channels in the body, promoting relaxation and focus.

- Kapalabhati (Skull Shining Breath): Energizes the body and improves digestion.

Meditation and Relaxation

- Mindfulness meditation: Cultivates present-moment awareness and reduces stress.

- Yoga Nidra: A deep relaxation technique that promotes physical and mental rejuvenation.

Tips for Beginners

- Start slowly: Begin with gentle poses and gradually increase the intensity.

- Find a qualified teacher: A qualified instructor can guide you through the poses and offer modifications.

- Regular practice: Consistency is key to experiencing the benefits of yoga.

- Listen to your body: Pay attention to your body's signals and avoid pushing yourself too hard.

By incorporating yoga into your routine, you can experience a significant boost in energy levels and overall well-being.

Pranayama, the practice of breath control, is a cornerstone of yoga. It can significantly impact energy levels, stress reduction, and overall well-being. Let's explore some effective techniques:

Energizing Pranayama Techniques

- **Kapalabhati (Skull Shining Breath): This technique is known for its energizing effects.**
  - Inhale deeply and forcefully exhale through the nose, using your abdominal muscles.
  - The exhalation should be short and powerful, while the inhalation is passive.
  - Begin with short bursts and gradually increase the duration.

- **Bhastrika (Bellows Breath): Similar to Kapalabhati, Bhastrika is also invigorating.**

  - Inhale and exhale forcefully through both nostrils, using the diaphragm.
  - The rhythm is faster than Kapalabhati.

- **Ujjayi Pranayama (Victorious Breath): This technique increases oxygen intake and calms the mind.**

  - Inhale and exhale through the nose, creating a gentle hissing sound.
  - The sound comes from the back of the throat.

Calming and Balancing Pranayama

- **Nadi Shodhana (Alternate Nostril Breathing): Balances the energy channels in the body.**
  - Close the right nostril with your right thumb and inhale through the left.
  - Close the left nostril with your ring finger and exhale through the right.
  - Continue alternating nostrils.

- **Sama Vritti (Equal Breathing): This technique promotes balance and relaxation.**

  - Inhale and exhale for the same count, maintaining a steady rhythm.

Important Considerations

- Practice regularly: Consistent practice is key to experiencing the benefits of pranayama.

- Start slowly: Begin with short sessions and gradually increase the duration.

- Listen to your body: Pay attention to your body's signals and avoid overexertion.

- Guidance: Consider learning from a qualified yoga teacher for proper technique.

Remember: Pranayama is a powerful tool, but it's essential to practice with awareness and respect for your body.

Meditation and mindfulness are powerful tools for managing chronic conditions like Chronic Fatigue Syndrome (CFS) and Fibromyalgia. By focusing on the present moment and calming the mind, these practices can help reduce stress, improve sleep, and enhance overall well-being.

Mindfulness Meditation

Mindfulness involves paying attention to the present moment without judgment. It helps to:

- Reduce stress: By focusing on the present, you can let go of worries about the past or future.

- Improve focus: Mindfulness can enhance concentration and attention span.

- Manage pain: By shifting attention away from pain, mindfulness can help reduce its intensity.

- Enhance sleep: Practicing mindfulness before bed can promote relaxation and better sleep.

Meditation Techniques

- Body scan: Focus attention on different parts of the body, noticing sensations without judgment.

- Breathing meditation: Concentrate on the rhythm of your breath, observing the inhale and exhale.

- Loving-kindness meditation: Cultivate feelings of warmth, kindness, and compassion towards yourself and others.

Incorporating Meditation into Daily Life

- Start small: Begin with short meditation sessions and gradually increase the duration.

- Find a quiet space: Create a peaceful environment for your meditation practice.

- Experiment with different techniques: Find what works best for you.

- Be patient: Meditation is a skill that takes time to develop.

Mindfulness in Daily Activities

Mindfulness can be practiced in any activity. For example:

- Mindful eating: Pay attention to the taste, texture, and smell of your food.

- Mindful walking: Focus on the sensations of your feet on the ground and the surrounding environment.

- Mindful showering: Notice the feel of the water on your skin and the sensations of your body.

By incorporating meditation and mindfulness into your daily life, you can significantly improve your quality of life and manage the challenges of CFS and Fibromyalgia.

Acupuncture and acupressure are complementary therapies rooted in Traditional Chinese Medicine (TCM) that have been used for centuries to treat various health conditions, including chronic pain.

Acupuncture

Acupuncture involves inserting thin needles into specific points on the body, known as acupoints. These points are believed to correspond to energy pathways (meridians). Stimulating these points is thought to regulate energy flow, promote healing, and relieve pain.

- Benefits for CFS and Fibromyalgia: Acupuncture may help reduce pain, improve sleep, and alleviate fatigue associated with these conditions.

- How it works: The exact mechanisms aren't fully understood, but it's believed to stimulate the release of endorphins and other neurotransmitters, reducing pain perception.

Acupressure

Similar to acupuncture, acupressure applies pressure to specific points on the body instead of needles. It's a self-treatment technique that can be easily learned and practiced at home.

- Benefits for CFS and Fibromyalgia: Acupressure can help alleviate pain, improve circulation, and promote relaxation.

- How it works: By applying pressure to acupoints, acupressure is believed to stimulate the body's natural healing processes.

Important Note: While acupuncture and acupressure can be beneficial for many people, it's essential to consult with a qualified practitioner to ensure safe and effective treatment.

Chiropractic Care for CFS and Fibromyalgia
Chiropractic care focuses on the musculoskeletal system, particularly the spine, and its relationship to overall health. It's based on the principle that the body has the innate ability to heal itself when the nervous system functions optimally.

How Chiropractic Care Can Help

- Pain reduction: By addressing misalignments in the spine, chiropractic adjustments can alleviate musculoskeletal pain often associated with CFS and fibromyalgia.

- Improved nervous system function: Correcting spinal imbalances can optimize nervous system function, potentially reducing symptoms.

- Enhanced sleep: Better spinal alignment can contribute to improved sleep quality, which is crucial for managing these conditions.

- Increased energy levels: By reducing pain and improving overall well-being, chiropractic care can help boost energy levels.

Chiropractic Techniques

Chiropractors use various techniques to adjust the spine and other joints, including:

- Spinal manipulation: Gentle, controlled adjustments to restore joint mobility.

- Mobilization: Gentle, rhythmic movements to improve joint flexibility.

- Soft tissue therapy: Massage and other techniques to relax muscles and reduce tension.

It's important to consult with a qualified chiropractor to determine if this approach is suitable for your specific condition.

Massage Therapy for CFS and Fibromyalgia
Massage therapy is a popular complementary therapy that involves manipulating the soft tissues of the body to promote relaxation, reduce pain, and improve circulation. It can be particularly beneficial for individuals with CFS and fibromyalgia.

Benefits of Massage Therapy

- Pain relief: Massage can help alleviate muscle tension and reduce pain associated with CFS and fibromyalgia.

- Improved circulation: Increased blood flow can help deliver oxygen and nutrients to the tissues, promoting healing.

- Stress reduction: Massage can induce relaxation and reduce stress levels, which can contribute to better sleep and overall well-being.

- Improved sleep: Regular massage can help regulate sleep patterns and improve sleep quality.

Types of Massage

There are various massage techniques that can be beneficial for CFS and fibromyalgia, including:

- Swedish massage: A gentle massage that focuses on relaxation and stress reduction.

- Deep tissue massage: Targets deeper layers of muscle tissue to release chronic tension.

- Trigger point therapy: Focuses on specific points of muscle tension to relieve pain.

It's essential to choose a massage therapist who is experienced in working with individuals with chronic conditions.

Relaxation techniques are essential for managing the stress and fatigue associated with CFS and fibromyalgia. These practices can help calm the mind, reduce muscle tension, and improve sleep quality.

Relaxation Techniques

- Progressive muscle relaxation: This technique involves tensing and releasing different muscle groups to promote relaxation.

- Guided imagery: This involves creating mental images of peaceful and relaxing scenes to reduce stress and anxiety.

- Hydrotherapy: Using water for relaxation, such as warm baths or showers, can soothe muscles and reduce pain.

- Yoga and tai chi: These gentle exercises combine physical movement with mindfulness, promoting relaxation and balance.

Incorporating Relaxation into Daily Life

- Create a relaxing environment: Designate a quiet space for relaxation.

- Practice regularly: Consistent practice is key to experiencing the benefits.

- Experiment with different techniques: Find what works best for you.

- Combine relaxation with other self-care practices: Incorporate relaxation into your overall wellness routine.

By incorporating relaxation techniques into your daily life, you can significantly improve your quality of life and manage the symptoms of CFS and fibromyalgia.

While we've covered several popular complementary therapies, there are many other options to explore. Here are a few more:

Mind-Body Therapies

- Hypnotherapy: This involves guided relaxation and focused concentration to achieve a trance-like state, allowing for therapeutic suggestions.

- Biofeedback: This technique provides information about physiological responses (like heart rate or muscle tension) to help individuals learn to control them.

Nutritional and Herbal Approaches

- Dietary changes: Certain dietary modifications, such as eliminating inflammatory foods or following specific diets (like the Mediterranean diet), may help manage symptoms.

- Supplements: Some supplements, like magnesium, vitamin D, or coenzyme Q10, are often explored for their potential benefits in CFS and fibromyalgia.

- Herbal remedies: Certain herbs, such as valerian root or St. John's wort, have been used to address specific symptoms.

Physical Therapies

- Pilates: This low-impact exercise focuses on core strength, flexibility, and posture, which can be beneficial for managing pain and fatigue.

- Water therapy: Exercises performed in water can reduce joint stress and improve mobility.

Important Considerations

- Consult with healthcare providers: Before starting any new therapy, it's essential to consult with your doctor or a qualified healthcare professional.

- Individualized approach: What works for one person may not work for another. It's important to find therapies that suit your individual needs and preferences.

- Combination therapies: Often, combining different therapies can provide the most significant benefits

.

Remember: While complementary therapies can be helpful, they should not replace conventional medical treatment. It's essential to work closely with your healthcare provider to develop a comprehensive treatment plan.a

Part IV: Coping and Support

Chronic Fatigue and Fibromyalgia: Impact on Daily Life
Chronic Fatigue Syndrome (CFS) and Fibromyalgia significantly impact daily life, affecting physical, emotional, and social well-being.

Physical Challenges

- Fatigue: Constant fatigue limits physical activity and daily routines.

- Pain: Widespread pain can hinder mobility and make simple tasks difficult.

- Sleep disturbances: Disrupted sleep exacerbates fatigue and affects overall functioning.

- Cognitive difficulties: Brain fog and difficulty concentrating impact work, study, and daily tasks.

Emotional Challenges

- Frustration: Dealing with limitations can lead to feelings of frustration and anger.

- Isolation: Reduced ability to participate in social activities can lead to loneliness.

- Depression and anxiety: These mental health conditions are common among those with CFS and fibromyalgia.

- Low self-esteem: Chronic illness can affect self-image and confidence.

Social Challenges

- Role changes: Adjusting to new roles within family and social circles.

- Relationship strains: Challenges in maintaining relationships due to reduced energy and availability.

- Employment difficulties: Difficulty holding a job or maintaining productivity.

- Financial strain: Medical expenses, reduced income, and increased costs due to illness can create financial challenges.

Coping Strategies

- Open communication: Discussing your challenges with loved ones can provide support and understanding.

- Setting realistic goals: Breaking down tasks into smaller, manageable steps can help prevent overwhelm.

- Time management: Prioritizing tasks and allowing for rest periods can help manage energy levels.

- Seeking support: Joining support groups or connecting with others facing similar challenges can provide emotional support.

Living with Chronic Fatigue Syndrome (CFS) or Fibromyalgia often involves significant adjustments to daily life. Here are some common challenges and strategies for coping:

Physical Challenges

- Reduced energy levels: Difficulty performing daily tasks, requiring adjustments in routines and expectations.

- Pain management: Finding effective ways to manage pain while maintaining daily activities.

- Sleep disturbances: Impact on daily functioning, mood, and energy levels.

Cognitive Challenges

- Brain fog: Difficulty concentrating, remembering details, and multitasking.

- Information overload: Struggling to process information and make decisions.

- Difficulty with multitasking: Needing to focus on one task at a time.

Social Challenges

- Isolation: Reduced ability to participate in social activities due to fatigue and pain.

- Relationship strains: Challenges in maintaining relationships due to changes in roles and responsibilities.

- Stigma: Dealing with misunderstandings and negative perceptions about the conditions.

Practical Adjustments

- Pacing activities: Balancing rest and activity to prevent overexertion.

- Creating a supportive environment: Making home adjustments for comfort and accessibility.

- Time management: Prioritizing tasks and allowing for rest periods.

- Seeking support: Building a support network of family, friends, or support groups.

- Adapting to changes: Accepting that daily routines may fluctuate and being flexible.

Emotional Challenges

- Frustration and anger: Dealing with limitations and setbacks.

- Depression and anxiety: Common emotional responses to chronic illness.

- Low self-esteem: Impact on self-image and confidence due to physical limitations.

Building a strong support system is essential for coping with the challenges of Chronic Fatigue Syndrome (CFS) and Fibromyalgia. Here are some valuable resources:

Support Groups

- Online communities: Connect with others facing similar challenges through online forums and support groups.

- Local support groups: Consider joining in-person support groups to build connections within your community.

- Peer-to-peer support: Sharing experiences with others can provide emotional support and practical advice.

Professional Support

- Healthcare providers: Maintain open communication with your doctors and specialists.

- Therapists: Seek support from mental health professionals to address emotional challenges.

- Social workers: Explore resources and assistance available through social services.

Practical Resources

- Advocacy organizations: Connect with organizations that advocate for the needs of individuals with CFS and fibromyalgia.

- Online information: Utilize reputable websites and resources for information and support.

- Accessibility services: Explore options for accommodations at work, school, or in the community.

Building a Strong Support Network

- Communicate openly: Share your challenges and needs with loved ones.

- Set boundaries: Establish realistic expectations and communicate your limitations.

- Seek support from unexpected sources: Explore support from colleagues, neighbors, or acquaintances.

- Online support communities: Utilize online platforms to connect with others.

By building a strong support network and utilizing available resources, individuals with CFS and fibromyalgia can better manage their conditions and improve their quality of life.

Open and honest communication with loved ones is essential for building understanding and support when living with CFS or Fibromyalgia. Here are some tips:

Expressing Your Needs

- Be clear and specific: Explain your symptoms and limitations in understandable terms.

- Set boundaries: Clearly communicate your needs and limitations without feeling guilty.

- Educate others: Provide information about CFS and Fibromyalgia to help them understand your condition.

Managing Expectations

- Be realistic: Avoid overpromising to prevent disappointment.

- Communicate fluctuating symptoms: Explain that your energy levels and pain may vary.

- Involve loved ones in decision-making: Include them in planning activities or making adjustments to daily routines.

Building Understanding

- Encourage empathy: Explain how the condition affects you emotionally and physically.

- Practice active listening: Allow loved ones to express their feelings and concerns.

- Show appreciation: Acknowledge their support and efforts.

Maintaining Connections

- Find alternative ways to connect: Explore activities that accommodate your energy levels, such as phone calls, video chats, or shared hobbies.

- Quality over quantity: Focus on meaningful interactions rather than frequent, tiring ones.

- Be patient with yourself and others: Understand that communication may be challenging at times.

Remember: Effective communication is a two-way street. It's important to listen to your loved ones' feelings and concerns as well.

Living with Chronic Fatigue Syndrome (CFS) or Fibromyalgia can be incredibly challenging. However, developing resilience and maintaining hope is crucial for navigating these difficulties.

Cultivating a Positive Mindset

- Focus on what you can control: Concentrate on areas where you can make a difference, such as self-care and managing symptoms.

- Practice gratitude: Recognizing and appreciating the positive aspects of your life can shift your perspective.

- Set realistic goals: Breaking down larger goals into smaller, achievable steps can boost confidence.

Building Resilience

- Embrace flexibility: Be open to adapting plans and routines as needed.

- Learn from setbacks: View challenges as opportunities for growth and learning.

- Build a support network: Connect with others who understand your experiences.

- Practice self-care: Prioritize activities that nurture your physical and emotional well-being.

Finding Meaning and Purpose

- Identify your values: Understanding what truly matters to you can provide direction and motivation.

- Contribute to others: Engaging in volunteer work or helping others can create a sense of purpose.

- Explore hobbies and interests: Discovering new passions can bring joy and fulfillment.

Seeking Professional Help

- Therapy: A therapist can provide tools and strategies for coping with challenges.

- Support groups: Connecting with others who understand your experiences can be invaluable.

- Medical professionals: Regular check-ins with healthcare providers can help manage symptoms and provide support.

Remember, building resilience is a journey, not a destination. It's important to be patient with yourself and celebrate small victories along the way.

Setting realistic goals is crucial for managing CFS and fibromyalgia. It helps to maintain motivation and prevent disappointment.

Understanding Realistic Goals

- Small, achievable steps: Break down larger goals into smaller, manageable tasks.

- Flexibility: Be prepared to adjust goals based on energy levels and symptom fluctuations.

- Focus on progress, not perfection: Celebrate small victories and avoid comparing yourself to others.

Creating SMART Goals

- Specific: Clearly define what you want to achieve.
- Measurable: Set goals that can be tracked and measured.
- Achievable: Ensure goals are within your capabilities.
- Relevant: Align goals with your overall well-being and priorities.
- Time-bound: Set a specific timeframe for achieving your goals.

Examples of Realistic Goals

- Physical goals: Increasing walking distance by 5 minutes each week.
- Mental goals: Practicing mindfulness for 10 minutes daily.
- Social goals: Attending one social event per month.
- Self-care goals: Taking a warm bath twice a week.

Celebrating Successes

- Recognize achievements: Acknowledge and reward yourself for reaching your goals.

- Learn from setbacks: Use challenges as opportunities for growth and adjustment.

Remember, the key to setting realistic goals is to listen to your body and avoid pushing yourself beyond your limits. By setting achievable goals and celebrating progress, you can build confidence and improve your overall well-being.

A strong support system is essential for individuals living with Chronic Fatigue Syndrome (CFS) or Fibromyalgia. It provides emotional support, practical assistance, and a sense of belonging.

Identifying Your Support Needs

- Emotional support: Sharing feelings and experiences with understanding individuals.

- Practical assistance: Help with daily tasks, errands, or childcare.

- Information and resources: Access to knowledge about the conditions and available support services.

- Companionship: Enjoying shared activities and social interactions.

Cultivating Existing Relationships

- Open communication: Share your challenges and needs with family and friends.

- Set boundaries: Establish clear expectations about the level of support you require.

- Quality time: Prioritize spending time with supportive loved ones.

Building New Connections

- Support groups: Join local or online support groups to connect with others facing similar challenges.

- Volunteer work: Engaging in activities that align with your interests can help build connections.

- Online communities: Utilize social media platforms to find support and connect with others.

Nurturing Your Support Network

- Gratitude: Express appreciation for the support you receive.
- Reciprocity: Offer support to others when possible.
- Quality over quantity: Focus on building deep connections with a few trusted individuals.
- Self-care: Prioritize your own well-being to maintain healthy relationships.

By investing time and effort in building a supportive community, you can enhance your overall well-being and cope more effectively with the challenges of CFS or Fibromyalgia.